THE ESTROGEN FREE® LIFESTYLE

THE ULTIMATE ESTROGEN DETOX

SECOND EDITION 2024

COPYRIGHT 2024 BY WENDY SELLENS BRONSON

ALL RIGHTS RESERVED. NO PART OF THIS PUBLICATION MAY BE REPRODUCED, DISTRIBUTED, OR TRANSMITTED IN ANY FORM OR BY ANY MEANS, INCLUDING PHOTOCOPYING, RECORDING, OR OTHER ELECTRONIC OR MECHANICAL METHODS, WITHOUT THE PRIOR WRITTEN PERMISSION OF THE AUTHOR, EXCEPT IN THE CASE OF BRIEF QUOTATIONS USED IN CRITICAL REVIEWS OR OTHER NON-COMMERCIAL USES PERMITTED BY COPYRIGHT LAW.

WENDY SELLENS BRONSON DACM LAC

Copyright © 2025 by Wendy Sellens Bronson DACM LAc

ISBN: 9798319248404

All rights reserved.

No part of this publication may be reproduced, distributed, or transmitted in any form or by any means, including photocopying, recording, or other electronic or mechanical methods, without the prior written permission of the publisher, except in the case of brief quotations embodied in critical reviews, and other noncommercial uses permitted by copyright law.

Medical editor "The Breast Thermography Revolution"
Brian Downum, LAc, MSTOM

Images provided by Pink Image Certified Breast Thermography
Wendy Sellens Bronson, LAc, DACM, and Martin Bales, LAc, DACM

TABLE OF CONTENTS

The Estrogen Lie
1

There is No Controversy - Only Physiology
2

What is Breast Thermography Research Proving?
3

Thermography
4

Estrogen Therapies Are Harmful
5

Estrogen Causes Estrogen Dominance
6

Excess Estrogen Causes Low Testosterone
7

Plants Have Hormones
8

Estrogen Causes PMS, Pain, Fibroids, & Dense Breasts
9

Estrogen Makes You Irritable & Causes Weight Gain
10

Estrogen Decreases Passion
11

Estrogen Causes Early Puberty & Infertility
12

The Estrogen Free® Lifestyle Level 1
13-28

The Estrogen Free® Lifestyle Level 2-5
29-35

Unlock the Secret to Permanent Hormone Balance
36

THE ESTROGEN FREE® LIFESTYLE

THE ESTROGEN LIE

This book comes with a warning: What you're about to learn may challenge everything you've been told about hormones. Be prepared to rethink your health and make powerful changes that could transform your life.

Prepare to be shocked—so shocked that your first instinct might be disbelief. The biggest lie women have been fed is that we are estrogen deficient! This little book will effortlessly guide you through the deceptions. You'll soon see just how pervasive estrogen is in our society and the havoc it has wreaked on every member of our families. Get ready, because this book is going to unfold like a soap opera—Welcome to the Days of Our Estrogen Lives.

Now, here's the good news! This is the simplest lifestyle change you'll ever make. Why? Because all you're doing is removing one hormone—the hormone responsible for estrogen dominance, PMS, menopause symptoms, infertility, weight gain, fibroids, PCOS, early puberty, and low testosterone, with an increased risk of breast cancer: Estrogen. If hormone specialists truly understood hormones, these disorders wouldn't be so widespread. You wouldn't be struggling or questioning, and I wouldn't be writing this book.

No health fads, no clever gimmicks, no essential oils needed, and let's stop the over-supplementing—you're just popping pills! It's time to stop spending hard-earned money and wasting precious time on yet another trend.

Remove the root cause- estrogen.

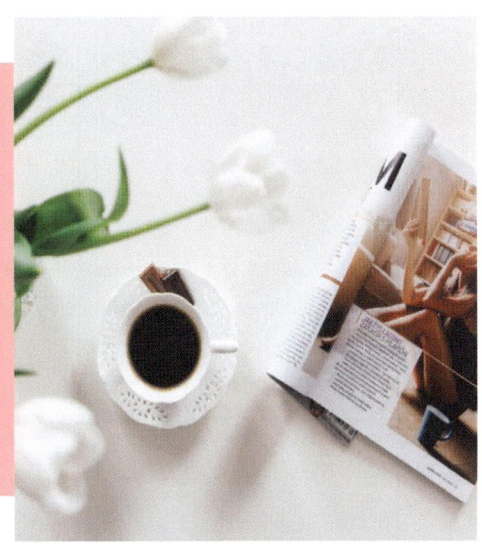

Let's get back to basics with a hormone-free life. The Estrogen Free® Lifestyle.

estrogen-free.com

THERE IS NO CONTROVERSY ONLY PHYSIOLOGY

This isn't just another diet—it's a lifestyle. A supplemental guide that seamlessly integrates into any diet or routine to help you reduce your risk from that notorious hormone: estrogen.

But here's the catch—estrogen is everywhere! It lurks in almost all processed foods, even organic ones. Many popular health fads and treatments are loaded with estrogen. Even organic or natural skincare products often contain estrogen as an ingredient. Shocked yet?

I'm going to guide you back to a simple, clean, hormone-free lifestyle! Using breast cancer statistics, physiology and medical evidence from breast thermograms. I'll show you what's really going on and what actually works.

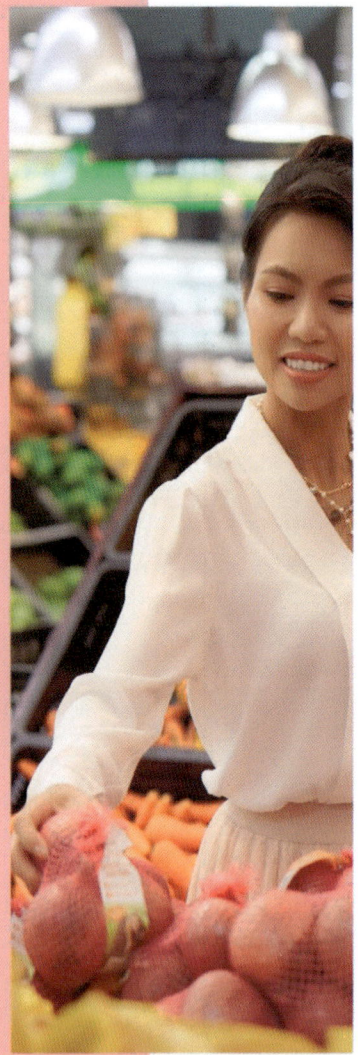

This book is an easy read for a complex issue. It's divided into two parts:

1. What estrogen is and what it does to your body
2. A 10-step guide to removing estrogens

Each section tackles a specific issue—read at your own pace. Let the information sink in, and then move on to the next step.

It's time to go back to school and educate ourselves! To fight a disease, you must understand how the disorder and your body work.

estrogen-free.com

WHAT IS BREAST THERMOGRAPHY RESEARCH PROVING?

Your blood vessels serve as an early warning system. Breast thermography evaluates the health of your breasts by monitoring these blood vessels. Cancers and other breast disorders, from benign masses to hormone imbalances like excess estrogen, often create specific patterns in the blood vessels. These vessels nourish and stimulate disorders, making thermography one of the first tools to identify potential issues. It's incredibly effective at detecting excess estrogen, also called progesterone deficiency in women, and testosterone deficiency in men, by observing the activity in the blood vessels.

In a "normal" thermogram, you won't "see" the blood vessels.

In an "at risk" or "abnormal" thermogram, the blood vessels become visible. It's that simple—anyone can "see" the difference with their own eyes.

Your breasts can't lie! Don't ignore the messenger that's trying to warn you. Just because this is new information doesn't mean it's incorrect—it's just new to you.

Breast thermography research is groundbreaking because it identifies what is beneficial or harmful to breast health before other imaging methods can. The key is our ability to "see" the blood vessels. It can take 6-10 years for breast cancer to be visible on a mammogram, meaning the cancer has been growing for several years. Thermography, however, can detect the early stimulation of blood vessels that may be feeding a disease or disorder long before other methods can.

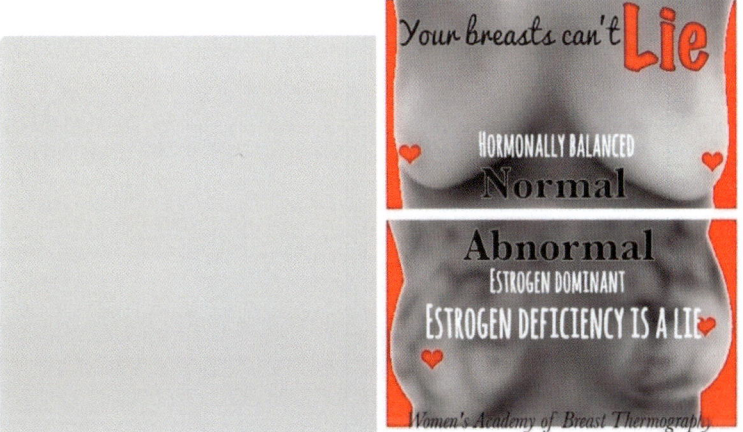

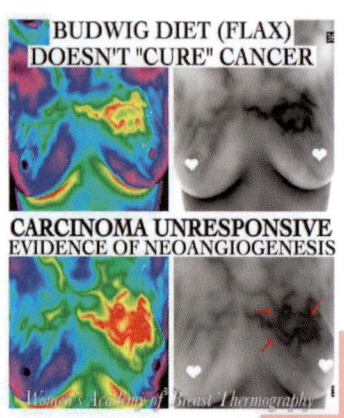

THERMOGRAPHY

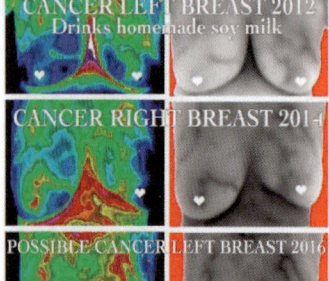

This is why our thermography research often uncovers medical evidence first—we can "see" changes in the blood vessels, whether good or bad, much earlier. We are the first line of defense, which is why our research is considered so radical. We publish and share our findings with other doctors, but change takes time.

Remember when everyone thought soy was safe? My mentor, Dr. Hobbins, was advising women to avoid soy—a plant estrogen—as far back as the '80s because it increased the risk of cancer and estrogen dominance.

Fifty years of breast thermography research has proven which therapies, herbs, supplements, and foods increase risk. What's truly amazing is that you can see small changes in the blood vessels in as little as 30 days. I can "test" whether a supplement is healthy or harmful. The blood vessels reveal if a treatment is effective and working, increasing risk, or if it's just a gimmick.

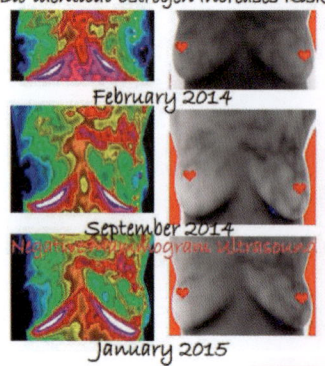

estrogen-free.com

ESTROGEN THERAPIES ARE HARMFUL

In traditional Chinese medicine, we are taught that the body is capable of living to 100-120 years. All that's required is a nutrient-rich, balanced diet. This is why your grandparents could smoke, drink, and still live to 95. In Chinese medicine, you visit the doctor to stay healthy. They use acupuncture treatments or herbal formulas to balance your body and maintain homeostasis. While they understand that the body will eventually age and die, they believe that by keeping it balanced, it will live healthier and longer.

In contrast, Western medicine often views the body as inherently weak and deficient. There's a prevailing belief that the body can't function properly without external aids like prescriptions and supplements. Many are familiar with the "God Complex" mentality, where the doctor is seen as the ultimate authority. In this system, the focus is often on treating symptoms rather than addressing the root cause, with an emphasis on pharmaceutical interventions. The body is frequently perceived as something that needs constant fixing, rather than something capable of natural balance and self-healing.

The body naturally produces the perfect amounts of healthy estrogen, progesterone, and testosterone tailored to each of us. Estrogen and progesterone are meant to be in balance—your body produces equal amounts of each. But when we start supplementing with estrogen, whether synthetic or plant-based, it disrupts this balance by raising estrogen levels and lowering progesterone and testosterone, leading to hormone imbalance.

Women have been misled by some doctors and the media into believing that estrogen therapy keeps us young and beautiful. This dangerous myth has cost thousands of mothers, daughters, and sisters their lives. Did you know that 80 percent of breast cancers are stimulated by estrogen? If we were truly estrogen deficient, breast cancer rates would be much lower. The rise in breast cancer began in the 1940s, coinciding with the introduction of estrogen therapy.

To heal, we must confront the hard truth. We need to stop buying into the propaganda designed to sell products and supplements. Thermographic research is showing that ALL forms of estrogen increase risk.

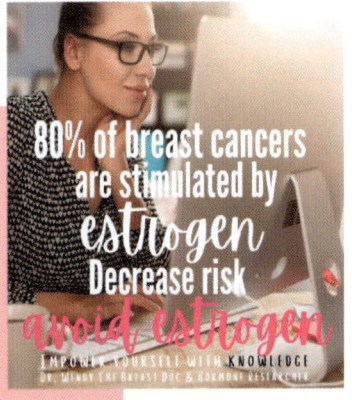

Our bodies are naturally designed to maintain balance and sustain life, a state known as homeostasis. This remarkable system doesn't require anything extra, such as supplements, to function.

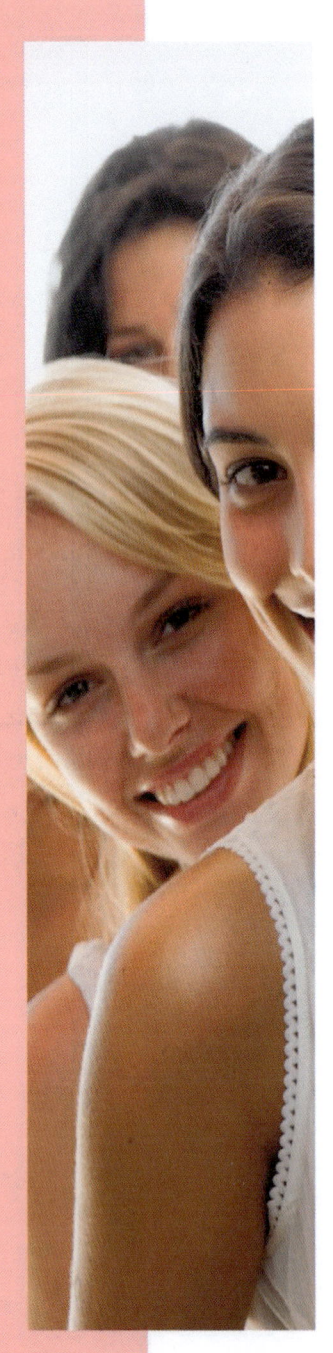

ESTROGEN CAUSES ESTROGEN DOMINANCE— OR MORE ACCURATELY PROGESTERONE DEFICIENCY

PMS and menopause symptoms are NOT normal! It's a disorder, a sign that you have excess estrogen or are progesterone deficient. Estrogen dominance is simply the result of overexposure to estrogen. Don't be misled by claims that it's due to impaired estrogen metabolism or liver function. These are myths that defy basic physiology and contribute to the rise in estrogen dominance, which I explore in depth in other books.

Signs and symptoms of excess estrogen typically include PMS, irregular or heavy periods, weight gain, hair loss, irritability, insomnia, anxiety, breast pain or itchiness, cramps, headaches, moodiness, bloating, nausea, fibrocystic and/or dense breasts, breast and uterine fibroids, endometriosis pain, and menopausal symptoms like hot flashes, night sweats, and low libido. Severe risks include infertility, thyroid issues, stroke, seizures, miscarriage, and breast and uterine cancer.

Here's another harsh truth: Estrogen therapy actually accelerates aging!

estrogen-free.com

EXCESS ESTROGEN CAUSES LOW TESTOSTERONE

It's time to "man up" and save the bros. Everyone is vulnerable to environmental estrogens, and for men, excess estrogen leads to low testosterone. What do you think causes Low T? It's a hormonal imbalance due to excess estrogen.

Symptoms of "Man-opause" include weight gain, infertility, low libido, erectile dysfunction, mood swings, depression, muscle weakness, reduced strength, hot flashes, decreased bone density, lower energy, motivation, memory/concentration issues, and loss of self-confidence. Sound familiar? These symptoms mirror what women experience on The Pill or during menopause.

While breast cancer in men is still considered rare, it's on the rise. Each year, about 2,000 new cases are expected in the U.S., with 400 men dying from the disease. The American Cancer Society reports that between 1975 and 2006, the incidence rate for men increased by 0.9 percent per year, with no clear explanation (not attributed to better detection).

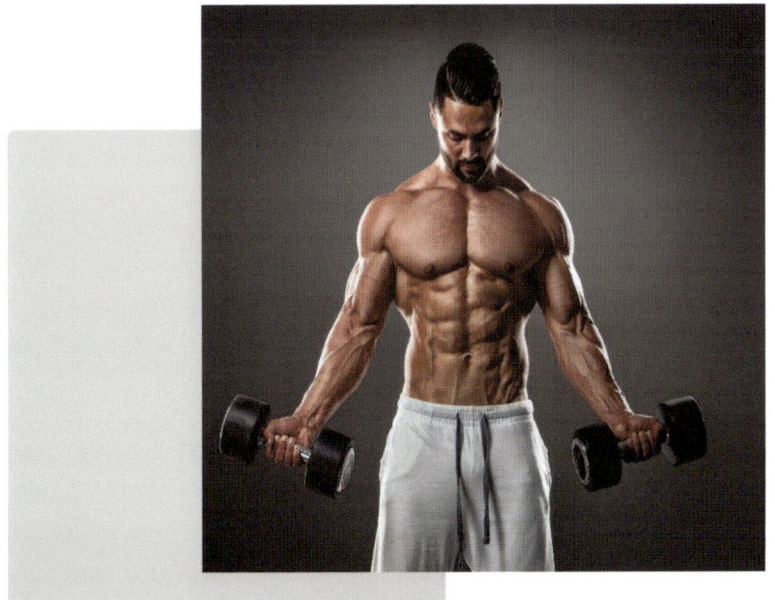

estrogen-free.com

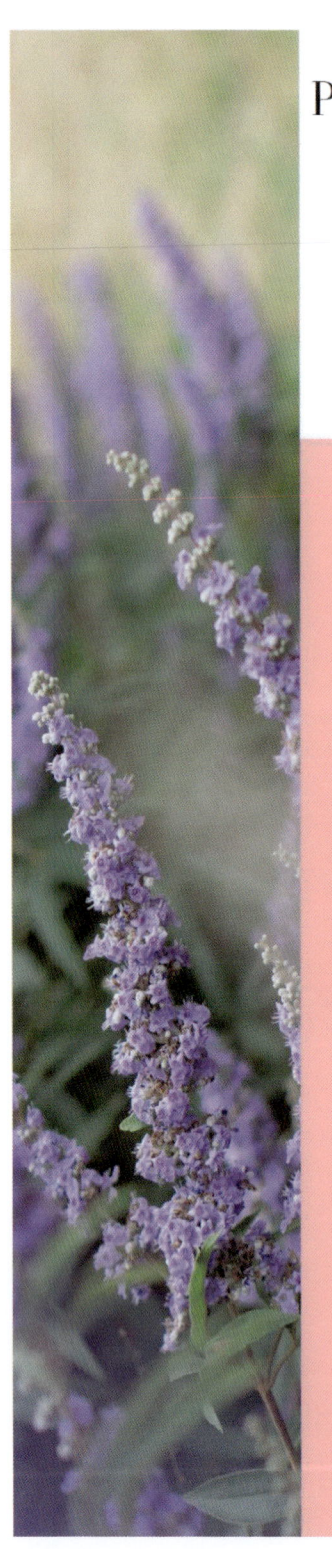

PLANTS HAVE HORMONES

One of the most surprising sources of estrogen is plant estrogens or phytoESTROGENS, often dismissed as weak or insignificant. But whether weak or not, they're still hormones, and plant estrogens have the same effect as any other: they bind and stimulate our receptors and raise estrogen levels in the body.

One of the most blatant lies out there is the medical myth that phytoestrogens block harmful estrogens. This is simply impossible. If a phytoestrogen can attach or bind to our receptors, it's stimulating them! If it can't attach, then it won't have any effect. This is basic physiology. Doctors claim phytoestrogens block estrogen, but then turn around and prescribe bio-identical estrogen, which is a phytoestrogen, wild yam. Do phytoestrogens block or treat? Which is it?

The term "bio-identical" doesn't mean safe or natural—it means similar chemical structure. Birth control pills, commercial-grade estrogens (xenoestrogens), flax, soy, even lavender, are all bio-identical, which is why they all contribute to excess estrogen.

You can't pick and choose, claiming one plant estrogen is harmful while another is safe. They all increase your risk. Be wary of these trendy, tricky terms designed to sell you DIS-ease.

ESTROGEN CAUSES PMS, PAIN, FIBROIDS, & DENSE BREASTS

Here's why: Estrogen is a powerful stimulator, causing blood vessels to engorge and become tense, leading to what we call dense breasts. Contrary to what we've been told, it's not the tissue itself—it's the blood vessels.

When the blood vessels are preparing for lactation, a normal physiologic response, they also expand or become tense, which causes the pain. It is the blood vessels that cause dense breasts from excess estrogen stimulation and is not normal. Pause...for the epiphany moment.

This explains why mammograms often struggle to provide accurate results when dealing with estrogen-induced density. When estrogen overstimulates the blood vessels, they expand, causing pain. Reduce your estrogen intake, and the pain should ease.

Estrogen also has a clotting factor, leading to breast and uterine masses. Side effects of birth control pills, such as heart attacks, pulmonary embolisms, and strokes, are all related to clotting disorders. If you have a history of fibroids or masses, it's crucial to avoid synthetic and plant estrogen—it will cause them to grow with continued use.

Doctors claim that synthetic estrogens and phytoestrogens don't cause these side effects, and that "studies" debunked this—False! Courts have proven that synthetic estrogen causes breast cancer, uterine cancer, heart attacks, pulmonary embolisms, and strokes, resulting in millions paid out to thousands of women. These estrogens are now required to carry warning labels on their packaging to alert all women to the risks.

What I'm trying to educate all women about is that the same side effects occur with phytoestrogens. This is proven by the fact that breast cancer remains the leading cancer among women, even as pharmaceutical sales of synthetic estrogen have significantly declined while bio-identical estrogen use has surged.

Many women are dealing with painful, dense breasts, which is treatable. Finally, you can find peace during your period!

ESTROGEN MAKES YOU IRRITABLE & CAUSES WEIGHT GAIN

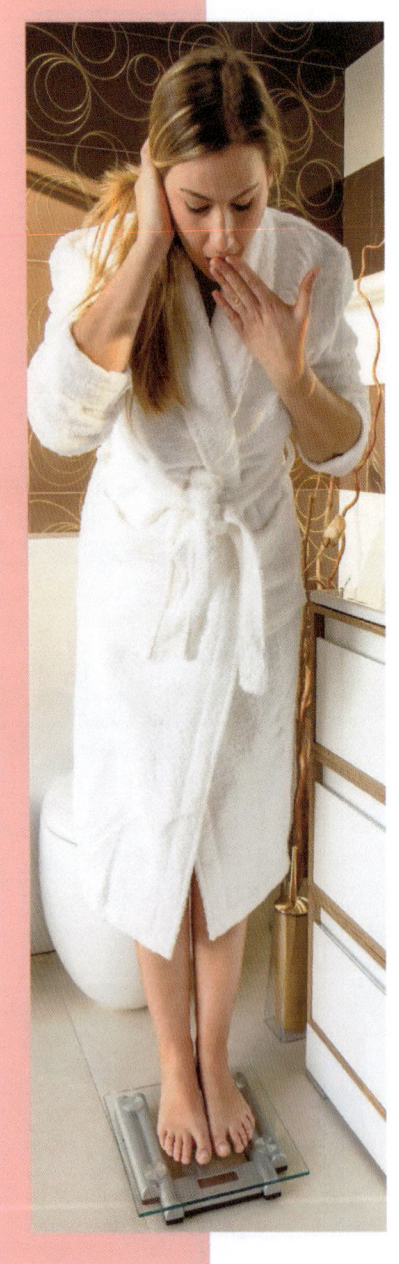

If estrogen therapies were as healthy as they claim, wouldn't they make you thin and Zen (calm)? This is why progesterone is sometimes required—to counteract the harmful effects of excess estrogen.

One of the most frustrating side effects of excess estrogen is irritability—but let's be real, it's more like feeling downright crazy! Tired of all the jokes? It's not cool when it feels like someone is squeezing our ovaries like a stress ball. Or worse, the week we turn into emotional whirlwinds—crying, yelling, and cranking the irritability up to 1,000—only to hear, "It must be your time of the month," which feels like a slap in the face! Sooo frustrating. But... how many times are they right?

The bitter truth is that "our time" often makes us irrational, unbearable, and impatient. To make matters worse, it can feel like we have no control, which only intensifies the situation. We barely recognize ourselves, and then we have to deal with the fallout of hurting those we love. And this vicious cycle repeats—monthly. But here's the sweet news, sisters! Estrogen is a stimulator, and when it's in excess, it causes irritability, anxiety, and insomnia. Achieving hormone balance equals finding your Zen.

You've heard about hormones used to fatten non-organic livestock, but did you ever wonder which one? Estrogen! Estrogen packs on the pounds! People who dive into health fads with flax or soy often notice weight gain but don't realize it's the estrogen, thinking they're being healthy. Calmness and weight loss are wonderful side effects of The Estrogen Free® Lifestyle!

ESTROGEN DECREASES PASSION

One unfortunate side effect of estrogen dominance is a decrease in passion for both men and women. Worse news – ever, huh? I've had many, many patients share with me their lack of libido and some report even an extreme feeling of what they call asexual. They often think they're the only ones going through this, but trust me, I hear it all the time. I understand how frustrating this can be, especially when it affects your relationship.

The good news? If you want to reignite your passion, it's simple—go estrogen free. Increasing your passion boosts intimacy, which strengthens your bond and deepens your relationship. Your partner will thank me—I love getting those messages!

Plus, research shows that cuddling, kissing, and sex reduce depression, stress, and pain, while improving sleep, immunity, muscle tone (yes, sex is cardio!), and releasing those feel-good hormones—endorphins and oxytocin.

Be Estrogen Free® and express your love!

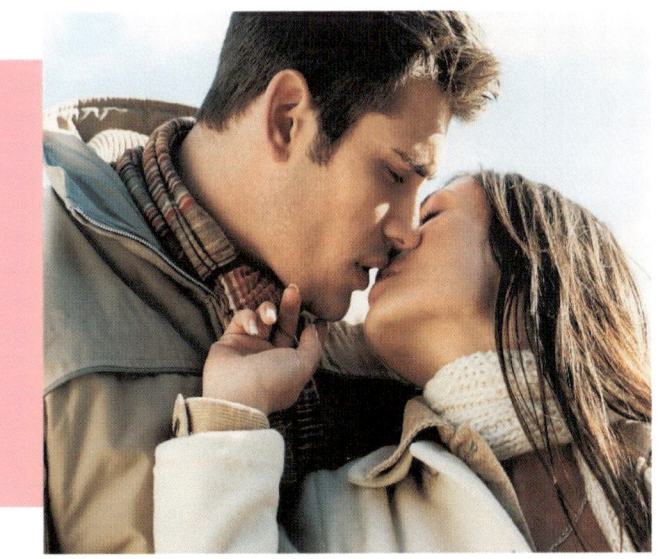

estrogen-free.com

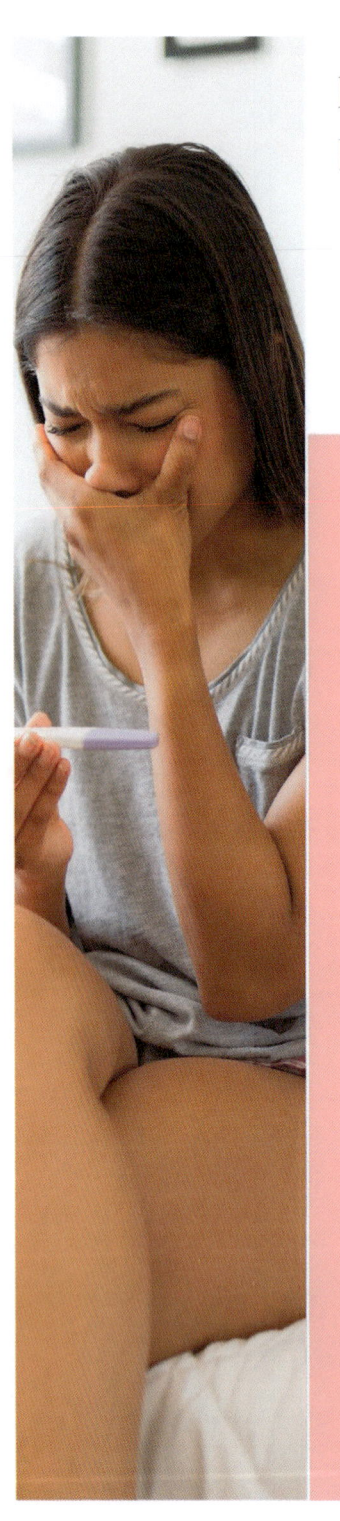

ESTROGEN CAUSES EARLY PUBERTY & INFERTILITY

Let's give kids back their youth. The hormones our bodies produce are healthy, but exposure to environmental estrogens in our food and household products are causing early puberty. America has the lowest average age of early puberty, starting at 8 years old, while in Europe, it begins at 9 years old.

A young girl's exposure to all types of estrogen will cause early puberty, including growth of breasts, early period; normal menarche is age 14-16. Other symptoms may include irregular or painful periods and breasts, depression, weight gain, hair loss, mood swings, anxiety, PCOS and possible infertility issues later.

For boys it may cause small organ size, mood swings, weight gain, muscle weakness, depression, low testosterone and possible sterility issues later.

Quick quiz – If you don't want to get pregnant, what do you do? Take The Pill. Why? Estrogen causes infertility. Now take this knowledge and translate it into your diet. Most of you immediately think, "Oh, hormones in chicken and beef." Correct. However, many of you may be using popular food products and trendy supplements thinking they are healthy, but they are causing infertility.

Stop being fooled by health fads.

estrogen-free.com

THE ESTROGEN FREE® LIFESTYLE

Building a new routine takes time, so don't overwhelm yourself or your family by trying to do everything at once. Some steps can be completed in a day, while others may take longer. Go at a pace that feels right for YOU. While some people can implement changes in a couple of weeks, it usually takes about 6 months to form a new habit.

Keep it simple. Use up your current products, and when it's time to shop, replace them with Estrogen Free® and chemical-free alternatives. This guidebook is short, concise, and packed with essential information, listing the estrogens you need to avoid, making it a practical and handy shopping companion—especially convenient in its ebook format for on-the-go reference.

There are three types of estrogen to avoid:
1. Commercial-grade estrogens are xenoestrogens or synthetic pseudo-estrogens, like pesticides, BPA, atrazine, phthalates, etc.
2. Plant estrogens or phytoestrogens.
3. Medical synthetic estrogens.

Stay informed. For a more detailed, routinely updated list as research progresses, visit the website: estrogen-free.com

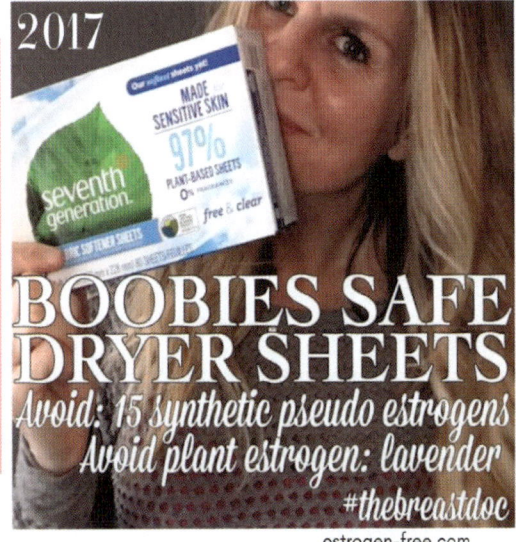

estrogen-free.com

STEP 1 ESTROGEN IN FOOD: FOOD IS YOUR DAILY MEDICINE

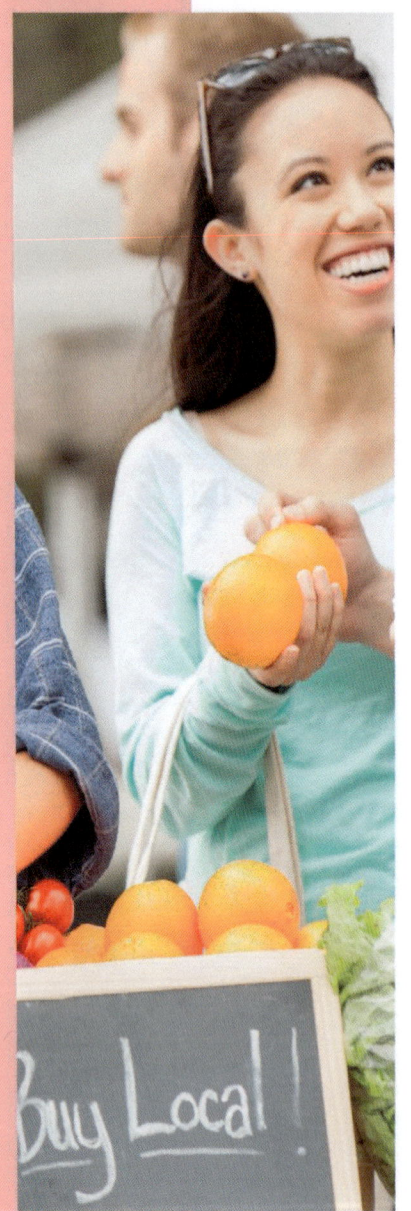

We hear a lot about hormones, but have you ever wondered which hormone is used to fatten conventional commercial livestock? It's estrogen! Estrogen causes weight gain, which is why it's the hormone of choice for fattening animals. Just ask anyone who has been on The Pill—they've likely noticed those extra pounds.

Grass-fed beef does not contain excess estrogen and won't raise your estrogen levels. This is plant-based propaganda. Throughout history, people have thrived on meat without hormonal issues.

When it comes to fruits and veggies, many pesticides and fertilizers contain xenoestrogens along with other chemicals.

Reduce your estrogen exposure by:
1. Start simple with - choosing higher quality or organic options at the store.
2. Buying directly from farmers at markets.
3. Start growing your own fruit and vegetables.

Remove all commercial-grade estrogens from your food:
- Avoid non-organic meats like beef, chicken, turkey, lamb, and pork.
- Avoid non-organic dairy products such as milk, cheese, sour cream, yogurt, and cottage cheese.
- Avoid non-organic fruits and vegetables. Whenever possible, buy straight from the farmer.

Don't end up like a fat cow pumped full of hormones—specifically estrogen.

Eating organic will significantly reduce your and your family's harmful exposure to environmental estrogens.

estrogen-free.com

STEP 1 ESTROGEN IN FOOD: YOU ARE WHAT YOU EAT

Just like people, animals are exposed to hormones through the plants they eat. If you consume chickens or turkeys that have been fed plant estrogens, you're also taking in those estrogens. This is similar to livestock given synthetic estrogen to fatten them up. Even when you pay more for organic meat or eggs, you could still be exposed to plant estrogens if their feed includes soy, flax or sesame.

When buying eggs or poultry, check the ingredients in their grain feed. Look for farmers or brands that avoid organic soy and flax.

Grass-fed beef and lamb are the healthiest choices. Remember, chickens are omnivores and eat everything from grain to bugs to mice.

Eggs are incredibly nutritious, especially the yolk, which is packed with nutrients. It contains healthy cholesterol, a precursor necessary for hormone production. Eating more eggs can help balance your hormones.

Avoid:
- Chickens, turkeys, and pigs fed plant estrogens, such as flax, sesame and soy, in their feed.

- Eggs labeled as omega-3, which usually means they contain flax.

- Fake foods (and people)! Fake cheese, fake milk, fake meat —they're loaded with high-estrogen ingredients, heavily processed, and often packed with sugar.

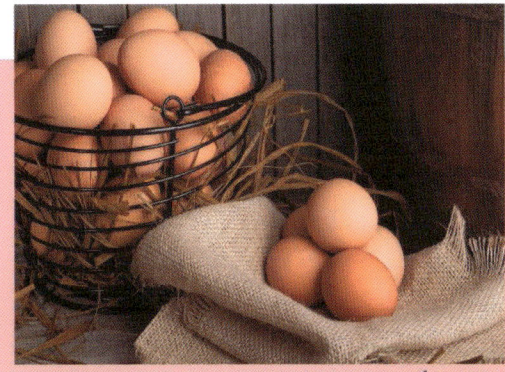

estrogen-free.com

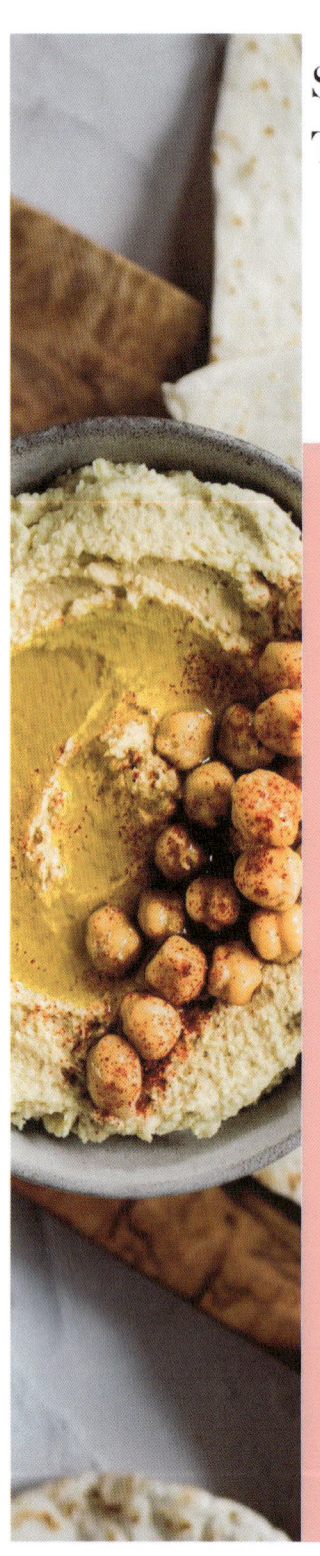

STEP 2
THE BIG 5 ESTROGENS

Most people are unknowingly consuming estrogen-laden foods because they're labeled as "healthy." Don't be fooled. Studies show that these phytoestrogens are among the strongest, with flax being 20 times more estrogenic than soy!

Flax is the new, more harmful soy. Nowadays, it's common knowledge that 1 cup of soy milk equals 1 birth control pill, but did you know that 1/4 cup of flaxseeds is equivalent to 20 birth control pills?

Don't be misled into thinking that organic flax or soy, whether in seed, oil, or cooked forms like tempeh, is safe or healthy—it's still a plant estrogen. You can't remove the hormone—estrogen—from the plant.

Take a look in your cupboards and check your ingredients. Most processed foods, even organic ones, use soy as an emulsifier. Soy is everywhere, and it's a major contributor to the rise in estrogen dominance across the board since the 1980s. Consumers have started demanding soy-free products, and now it's time to ditch flax and the other Big 5 estrogens, too!

Avoid The Big 5:
- Flax – oil, seeds, crackers, chips, cereal, and milk
- Soy – tofu, edamame, fermented soy, cereal, milk, cheese, and meats
- Garbanzo beans, or chickpeas - hummus, pasta and chips
- Sesame – oil, crackers, or bread
- Multigrain or powerseed – breads, crackers, and cereals containing rye, soy, flax, and sesame

estrogen-free.com

STEP 3 ESTROGEN IN WATER: PURE WATER

Did you know that your filtered water might contain hormones? Yes, you could be drinking everyone's Prozac, Lipitor, and more crucially for your hormone balance, HRTs (hormone replacement therapy) and BCPs (birth control pills). And to make matters worse, most "filtered" water is stored in plastic bottles containing BPA, a synthetic estrogen. To remove medical waste, microplastics, and hormones from your water, you need a special filter. The filter must be at least 1/10,000 of a micron to ensure optimal quality. Unfortunately, this level of filtration is no longer available on the market. This filter not only removes contaminants but also alkalizes your water, just as nature intended, while providing your daily supply of essential minerals—no need for extra supplements. Get magnesium from your water, just as Mother Nature meant it to be.

Avoid these types of water that may contain synthetic pseudo-estrogens, plastics, BPA, pesticides, and possible pharmaceuticals:
- Filtered water (e.g., Brita, Pur)
- Bottled water
- Reverse osmosis filtration

Drink real water as nature intended.

For more information, read the blog: "Drink it up! 5 Reasons Why Your Alkaline Water Isn't Hydrating You & Is Loaded With Hormones" at abreastboutique.com

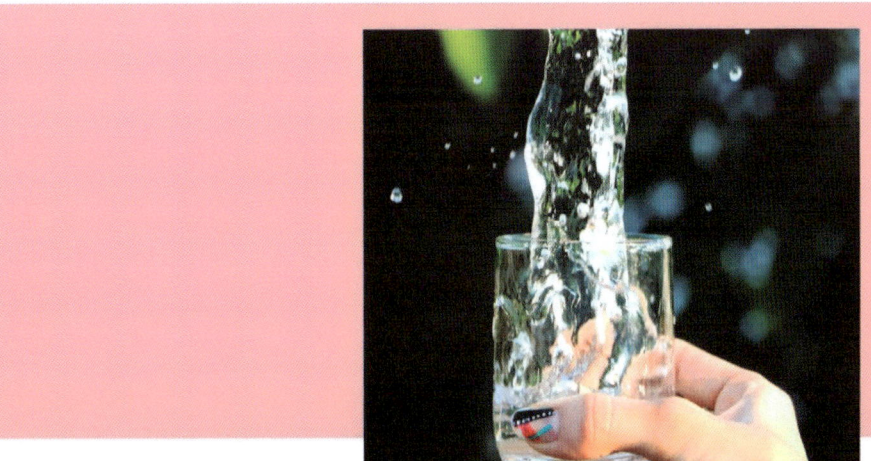

estrogen-free.com

STEP 4 ESTROGEN IN DRINKS: NO NEED TO W(H)INE, COFFEE & TEA ARE FINE

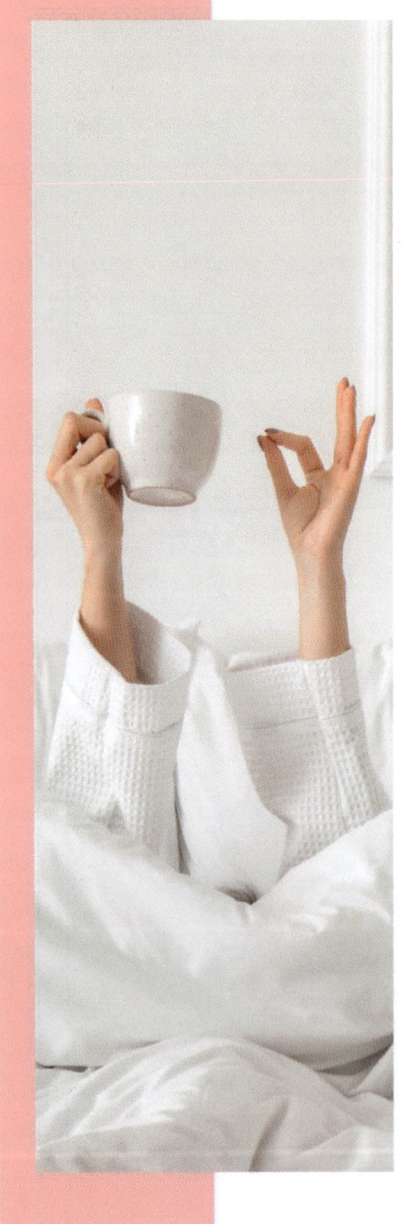

Get ready for a surprise: coffee actually contains less plant estrogen than green tea. So why does coffee get such a bad rap? Coffee doesn't cause fibroids or breast cancer; however, it is one of the most heavily sprayed crops, and those chemicals are concentrated into a single cup. The real question is, what is causing the fibroids and cancer risk? Organic coffee, especially on a Monday morning, is a girl's best friend! In moderation, coffee and tea are high in antioxidants, boost metabolism, and are natural stimulants. This blog focuses exclusively on hormones, but there are other experts discussing topics like mold and more.

Cheers! Hops, found in beer, is a plant estrogen, and so is resveratrol, an ingredient in red wine. I know mama needs to w(h)ine, so try—yes, try—switching to organic white wine, champagne, and organic spirits, including tequila. Drink less beer and red wine, or enjoy them only as needed—wink wink. Remember, being happy is healthy! Some ladies need their cheat days!

There's also a lot of misinformation about milk. If you want to drink milk, let's get the facts straight. Real milk, straight from the cow, known as raw milk, doesn't contain estrogen because cows aren't producing estrogen when they're nursing. Raw, nutrient-dense milk really "does the body good." More importantly, pasteurization causes inflammation, so choose wisely!

Avoid:
- Non-organic tea and coffee
- Tea bags due to chemicals
- Non-organic pasteurized, homogenized milk
- Excessive hops and resveratrol

STEP 5 ESTROGEN IN SUPPLEMENTS: DON'T BE A PILL (OR POWDER) POPPER

You can't supplement your way to a healthy life. Many supplements are either not bioavailable or, even worse, contain estrogen. Be cautious with popular women's or breast supplements, creams, or oils—most contain estrogen. Ironically, the very treatments meant to address hormone imbalances are often causing them!

Avoid popular products that start with "Est," "Meno," "Phyto," or "Women's"—they often contain phytoestrogens. Examples include bio-identical estrogen pellets, patches, and creams, Estrovera (rhubarb root), Estrovite (black cohosh), Essiac Tea (burdock root), Hoxsey Tonic (licorice, red clover, burdock root), Myomin (xiang fu), and Wild Yam.

"Natural" estrogen blockers might sound effective, but they don't work. After monitoring breast cancer patients with thermography for sixteen years, I have never seen a decrease in vascularity or risk with these products. In fact, many of them actually increase risk. Avoid products including Chinese herbal formulas containing xiang fu, dong quai, and pu gong ying, as these are all phytoestrogens, unless perscribed by a Chinese medical doctor.

By living Estrogen Free®, you naturally reduce your estrogen levels—there's no need for blockers. Simply stop using what's causing the problem: estrogen. Some patients may choose to raise their low progesterone and testosterone levels, which can be effective and finally create hormone balance, or as I like to call it, hormone bliss.

Remove estrogen
Ashwagandha, Flax, Sesame, Chick pea, CBD, Milk thistle, Licorice, Soy, Hemp, Astragalus, Primrose, Rhubarb, Turmeric, Red clover, Lavender, Chasteberry/Vitex, Black cohosh

DR. WENDY THE BREAST DOC & HORMONE RESEARCHER

estrogen-free.com

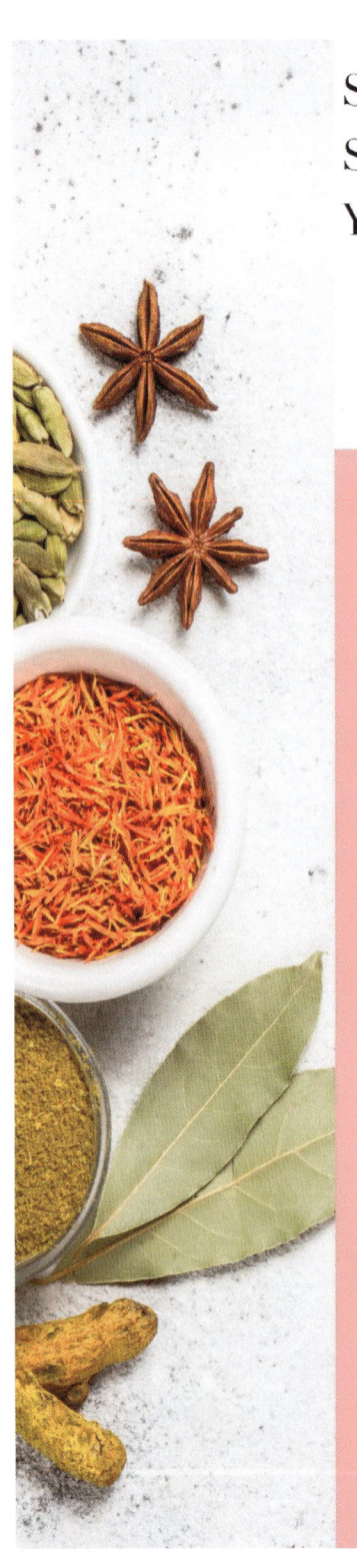

STEP 5 ESTROGEN IN SUPPLEMENTS: CUSTOMIZE YOUR SUPPLEMENTS FOR YOU

Avoid using trendy herbs unless prescribed by a professional. Herbs are powerful medicines with potential contraindications and side effects. In Chinese medicine, a single herb is rarely prescribed on its own. Instead, an herbal formula is customized for each individual, treating the whole body rather than relying on multiple bottles of pills. Herbs work synergistically—they enhance each other's strengths, reduce toxicity, or mitigate unwanted side effects. What works for one person might not work for another and could even cause an imbalance or worse. An experienced herbalist has spent years mastering these interactions and, most importantly, ensuring they do no harm.

Only use these organic herbs as needed for short-term treatment, as long-term use can increase estrogen dominance:
- Ashwagandha/Indian ginseng
- Asian ginseng • Astragalus/Huang qi
- Black Cohosh
- Burdock root
- CBD & Hemp
- Chasteberry/Vitex
- Dong Gui/Dong Quai
- Fo-Ti/Ye Jiao Teng
- Kudzu root
- Licorice
- North American ginseng
- Milk thistle
- Mistletoe
- Red Clover
- Resveratrol
- Rhubarb
- Turmeric
- Xiang Fu

Be holistic. Seek out a qualified Traditional Chinese medical herbalist who can prescribe a herbal formula tailored just for you.

STEP 5 ESTROGEN IN SUPPLEMENTS: THE BIG OIL SPILL

This section may come as a surprise to all the Mommy Bosses excited about the essential oil craze and home businesses. Essential oils work because plants are powerful, but remember—essential oils are highly concentrated and, like herbs, they are medicine. It's important to respect both plants and essential oils. Avoid applying them directly to the skin or ingesting them daily, or even weekly. Use them only as a short-term treatment.

Warning: Do not use essential oils on children, pregnant, or lactating women. If necessary, for a child always dilute them and use short term. Breast cancer patients need to avoid, too.

Avoid these concentrated organic estrogenic essential oils:
- Lavender
- Aniseed
- Basil
- Chamomile
- Cinnamon
- Clary Sage
- Coriander
- Cypress
- Evening Primrose
- Fennel
- Geranium
- Oregano
- Peppermint
- Rose
- Rosemary
- Sage
- Tea Tree
- Thyme

This complex topic can't be covered briefly, so it's explored in depth in books and frequently discussed on social media.

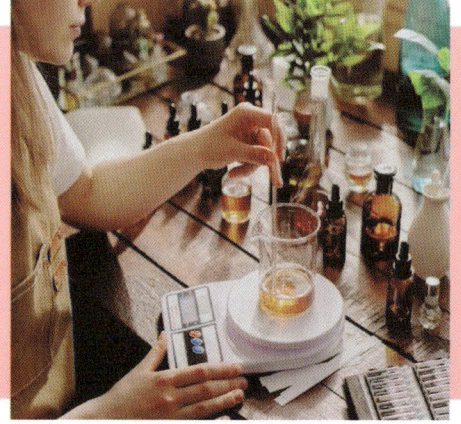

Including fresh herbs in your meals or teas as part of a balanced diet is both healthy and highly encouraged!

estrogen-free.com

STEP 6 ESTROGEN IN SKINCARE: NATURAL BEAUTIES

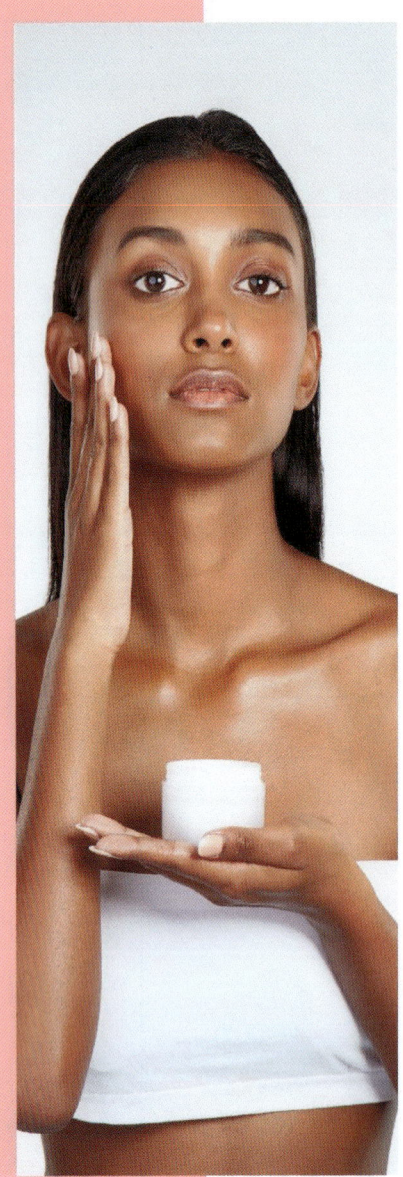

Everything you rub, buff, or massage onto your skin is absorbed into your bloodstream. Conventional skincare products increase your exposure to synthetic estrogens, contributing to excess estrogen in the entire family.

Just as you consider what you eat, it's crucial to think about what your skin absorbs. The estrogen, BPA, parabens, and lavender in deodorants and lotions are known to increase health risks. It's time to ditch those toxic products, especially breast products or "boobie butters."

Stick with clean, safe, unscented bases like coconut, shea, avacado and jojoba.

Avoid synthetic pseudo estrogens:
- Sulfates
- Parabens (propylparaben, butylparaben)
- Phthalates
- Triclosan
- Petroleum

Avoid hormone estrogenic bases and scents in popular organic, natural or chemical-free skincare products:
- Hemp or CBD
- Lavender
- Rose
- Geranium
- Peppermint
- Tea tree
- Etc

Avoid toxic heavy metals:
- Aluminum

estrogen-free.com

STEP 7 ESTROGEN IN PERIOD PRODUCTS: SAVE THE V

Oooh la la, organic cotton! For years, we've unknowingly exposed ourselves to harmful chemicals through the vagina, which is highly porous and absorbs substances quickly and efficiently. Conventional tampons are loaded with synthetic estrogens and chemicals like chlorine, dioxin, rayon, pesticides, dyes, and fragrances. These toxic ingredients can cause cancer, toxic shock syndrome, reproductive issues, and hormone disruptions—specifically estrogen dominance from synthetic estrogens.

Treat your vagina like the delicate flower it is. Avoid estrogen creams; the vagina is a muscle, and estrogen doesn't treat muscles. Do you use estrogen for a muscle tear? No. Many women who complain of vaginal dryness are actually estrogen dominant—estrogen isn't the solution!

Protect your vagina, sisters! Period. If you make only one change, make it this one: switch to organic tampons or pads.

Avoid:
- Conventional pads, panty liners, and tampons
- Scented products
- Estrogen creams

Clean ingredients for a clean V.

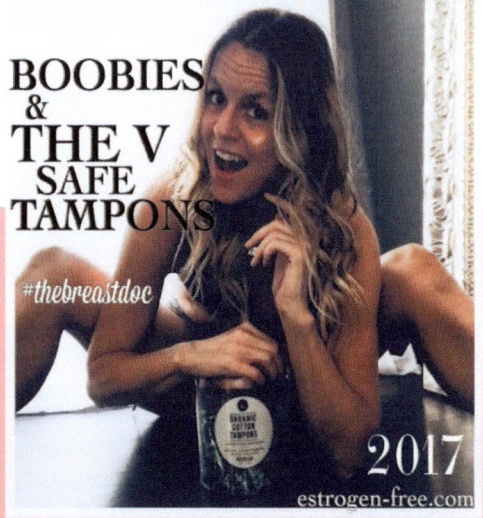

estrogen-free.com

STEP 7 SILICONE MENSTRUAL CUPS: A MODERN ALTERNATIVE WITH CAUTION

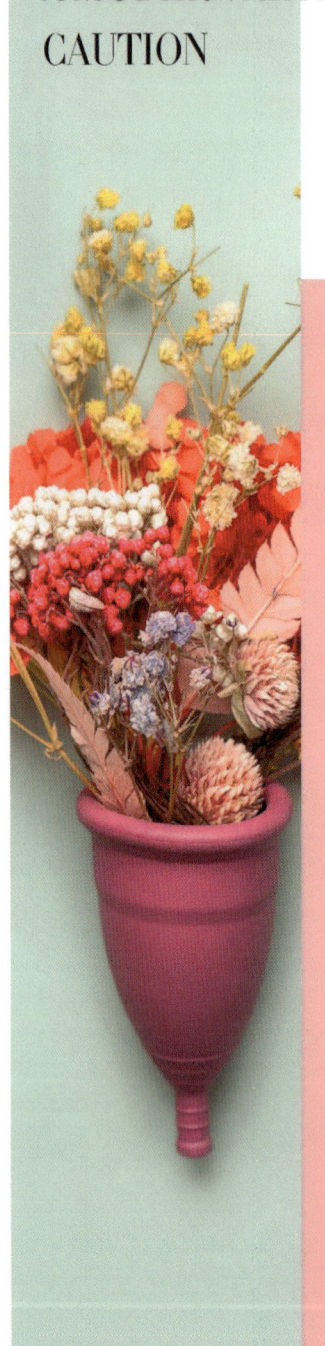

Silicone menstrual cups, often marketed as a sustainable and convenient alternative to tampons and pads, have gained popularity for their eco-friendly appeal. Made from medical-grade silicone, these cups are designed to be reusable, reducing waste and saving money over time. However, while they may seem like a perfect solution, it's important to approach their use with caution.

Considerations:
• Chemical Exposure: Silicone is a synthetic material, and while medical-grade silicone is generally considered safe, it's still important to be mindful of potential chemical exposure. Over time, repeated use can lead to wear and tear, potentially releasing small amounts of silicone into the body.

• Hygiene and Maintenance: Proper hygiene is crucial when using menstrual cups. They need to be thoroughly cleaned and sterilized between uses to prevent bacterial growth, which can lead to infections if not handled correctly.

• Fit and Comfort: Not all menstrual cups are created equal, and finding the right fit can be a trial-and-error process. An ill-fitting cup can cause discomfort, leakage, or even disrupt the natural balance of the vaginal flora.

• Long-Term Use: While menstrual cups can be a great option for many, it's important to monitor how your body responds to their long-term use. Pay attention to any changes in comfort or health, and don't hesitate to switch to another product if needed.

While silicone menstrual cups offer a modern and environmentally friendly alternative, it's essential to use them with care and stay aware of your body's needs. As with any product, what works well for one person might not be the best choice for another.

estrogen-free.com

STEP 8 ESTROGEN IN SOAP: SUPER DUPER SANITIZED

Refreshingly real! That squeaky clean feeling from conventional soap loaded with chemicals? It's actually stripping your skin of its natural protective barrier, leading to dryness and potentially acne. Real soap, combined with warm water and a bit of friction, is all you need to stay clean—tried and tested for generations before chemical cleaning agents were even a thing. When it comes to hair care, it's about nourishment and strengthening.

Chemicals can strip your hair, leaving it dry, flat, frizzy, and may even fade color. Luckily, there are now some incredible products available that deliver pure gorgeousness without the harmful chemicals.

Avoid:
• Xenoestrogens such as parabens (propylparaben, butylparaben), phthalates, Triclosan.
• Plant estrogens like lavender, rosemary, rose, peppermint, aloe, and tea tree in organic soaps, shampoos, and conditioners.
Your skin will love getting back to basics with real soap.

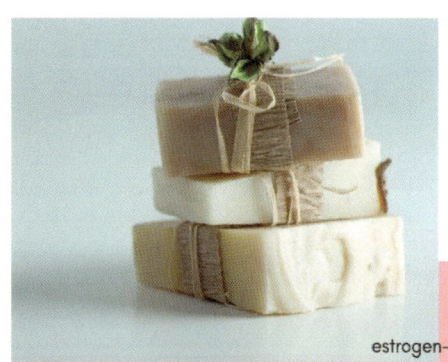

Ever wonder why diseases and disorders are on the rise? One factor is transgenerational exposure—mothers passing the chemicals in their bodies to their children. Each generation becomes weaker, carrying more chemicals and potential genetic disorders, while bacteria mutate and grow stronger. For the sake of future generations and mother earth, it's time to stop using harmful chemicals and estrogen.

Triclosan is another. Let's call it what it is—a synthetic estrogen. It's even in hand sanitizers and wipes, which many moms are using multiple times daily on their kids! Soap has been effective for thousands of years—let's go back to basics.

What's interesting is that while doctors no longer hand out antibiotics like candy, they still recommend hand sanitizers—which are a form of antibiotic! Even in smaller doses, used every day, multiple times a day, the effects accumulate. Throw it out. Stop sanitizing your house and family with anti-bacterial cleaners. Over-sanitization weakens your immune system, making you more susceptible to everyday bacteria, leading to allergies and hypersensitivity.

Avoid:
• Hand sanitizers, anti-bacterial soaps, and cleaners labeled "anti-bac."
• Toxic household cleaners containing petrochemicals, which are xenoestrogens.
• Estrogenic essential oils like lavender and geranium; citrus is usually a safer scent.

estrogen-free.com

STEP 8 ESTROGEN IN LAUNDRY SOAP: SNUGGLE UP TO CLEAN

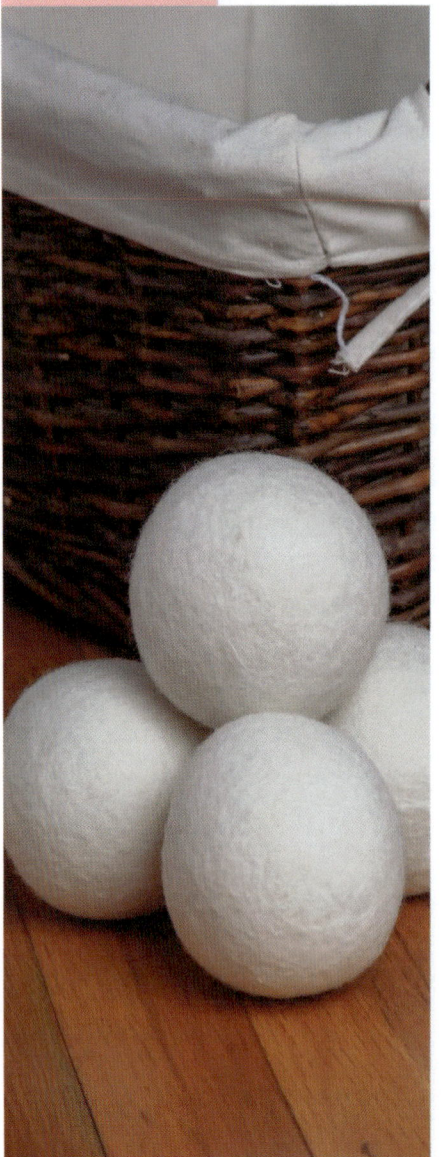

The pure smell of clean. It's reported that the typical American home contains 3-10 gallons of toxic products, with the EPA noting that indoor air can be 2-5 times more polluted than outdoor air due to common household products. Researchers have found that dryer sheets and air fresheners contain some of the highest concentrations of chemicals among all household products tested. Since dryer sheets are classified as cleaners, the EPA does not require testing or ingredient disclosure.

Dryer sheets are one of the most harmful household products for two reasons: First, the chemical film they leave behind is absorbed through the skin, with these chemicals and synthetic estrogens being stored in fat cells, contributing to estrogen dominance. Second, the synthetic fragrances are not only carcinogenic but also pollute our air, causing respiratory diseases and disorders.

Avoid this scary laundry list:
• Detergents containing sodium lauryl sulfate (a carcinogenic synthetic estrogen), NPE (nonylphenol ethoxylate, another xenoestrogens), 1,4-dioxane (carcinogenic), and phosphates (skin irritants).
• Dryer sheets, which can contain up to 15 synthetic estrogens.

Instead, use wool balls or chemical and Estrogen Free® dryer sheets.

estrogen-free.com

STEP 9 COMMERCIAL GRADE ESTROGENS: TOXICITY EXPOSED

Bye bye, plastic! You've spent your hard-earned money on hormone-free food, so why cook and store it in chemical-laden products? Avoid plastic—and yes, even BPA-free products. We all know BPA contains a synthetic estrogen, but BPA-free products often contain BSA, which has recently been found to be toxic as well.

All petrochemical products contain xenoestrogens, or commercial-grade estrogens, which raise estrogen levels in your body. Stick with glass, wood, and stainless steel, especially when freezing or heating food. Avoid cooking with plastic, rubber spatulas, and kitchen appliances made of plastic, like coffee makers, as these materials can transfer chemicals to your food when heated.

Avoid:
- BPA-free and BSA containers
- Rubber or plastic cooking materials—spatulas, coffee makers
- Canned food—BPA in the lining
- Plastic—don't freeze or heat plastic items like ice cube trays, bottles, cups, Tupperware, and bowls

The little chemicals you never think about:
- Teflon skillets, pans, grills and waffle makers
- Heating Styrofoam or pouring hot liquid into Styrofoam
- Off-gassing from new furniture, carpet, and clothes
- Paints, household cleaners, and fuel

> Stop, stop, stop cooking with plastic and drinking out of plastic!

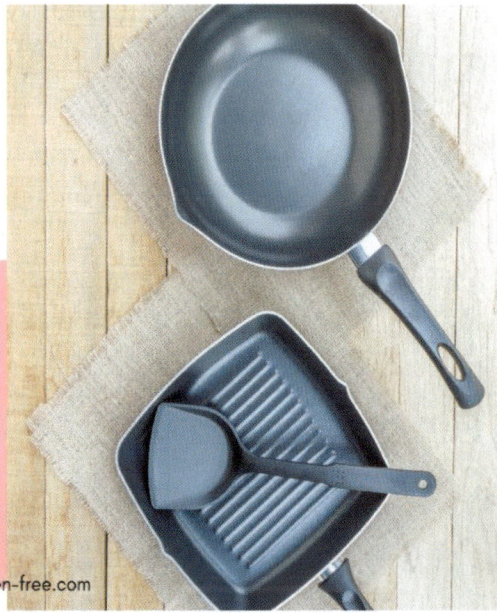

estrogen-free.com

STEP 10 SYNTHETIC ESTROGEN: OUR MOTHERS WERE LAB RATS

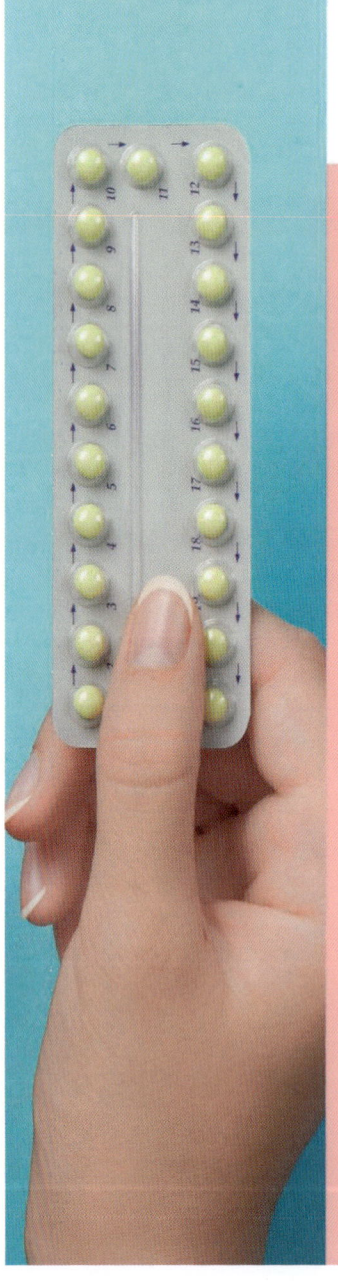

The statistics on pharmaceutical-grade synthetic estrogen are shocking! These are the most harmful forms of estrogen. Anyone who has tried to get birth control pills (The Pill) or hormone replacement therapy (HRTs) knows that you have to sign a waiver acknowledging the severe side effects—breast cancer, uterine cancer, stroke, heart attack, seizures, and DVTs. There are countless lawsuits involving estrogen therapies, and I strongly encourage you to research your specific brand and see the side effects for yourself. Mind blown!

The Pill increases your risk of breast cancer by four times. Estrogen shots are contributing to rising sterility rates. One of the largest studies on HRTs, initially believed to uncover the fountain of youth, instead revealed a dramatic increase in the very side effects mentioned above.

Avoid:
- Hormone replacement therapy (HRTs)
- Birth control pills (BCPs)
- Hormonal IUDs
- Estrogen injections, patches, vaginal rings, and creams

The safest contraceptive options are copper IUDs or chemical-free condoms. Save yourself—make the switch.

Now, they're trying to convince us to use bio-identical estrogen, once again without any studies proving its efficacy. I was the first researcher to publish medical evidence showing that bio identical estrogen increases risk. Avoid bio-identical estrogen products also called wild yam cream.

Don't become a story in one of my books!

estrogen-free.com

THE ESTROGEN FREE® LIFESTYLE LEVEL 2-5

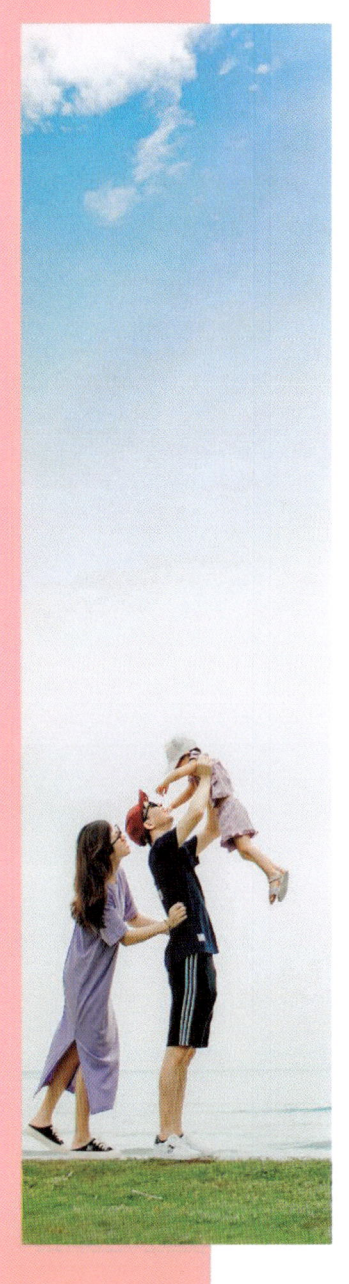

Life is meant to be savored and enjoyed. The recommendations provided here are intended to help you minimize your exposure to estrogen. However, it's important to remember that it's okay to have a cheat day when needed. Life is all about finding balance – there are days for eating healthy, and then there are days to indulge in cookies.

It is unrealistic to aim for the complete elimination of all estrogens from your environment because fruits, vegetables, seeds and beans contain phytoestrogens. The only true Estrogen Free Diet would be carnivore. Therefore, the concept of balance, or ratio, becomes crucial in managing estrogen exposure. The strategy involves removing synthetic estrogens and potent phytoestrogens from your routine, allowing for the occasional use of weaker phytoestrogenic substances. This approach is particularly relevant if you need to treat certain health conditions with phytoestrogenic herbs or if you choose to use products occasionally that contain one or two weak phytoestrogen, such as sage.

Strive to live naturally. Don't be overwhelmed by this list.

Start with Level 1, which is highly effective, and consider this additional information as you progress on your journey to a healthier lifestyle.

estrogen-free.com

LEVEL 2

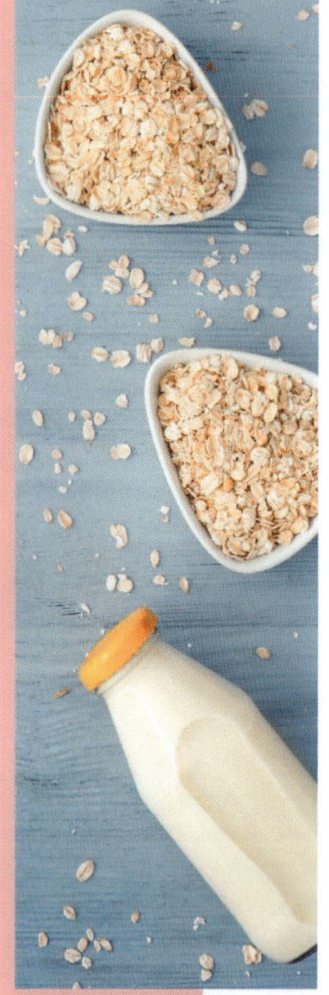

Rather than discarding food and household items immediately, you may want to consider using them and then opting for Estrogen Free® foods and products when it's time to replace them.

Avoid Estrogenic Seed Oils:
- Sunflower oil
- Peanut oil

Only consume "first cold press" olive oil without overheating, which can potentially make it rancid.

Avoid Estrogenic Fake Milks:
- Organic flax milk
- Organic oat milk
- Organic almond milk
- Organic soy milk

Avoid Adaptogens:
- Ginseng
- Ashwagandha
- Golden root
- Holy Basil

Avoid Plastic and BPA. BPA-free, including Alternatives BPS, BPAF, and TMBPF:
- Bottled water
- Tap water
- Brita or similar filtered water containers
- Plastic food and drink containers
- Plastic sippy cups
- Plastic in the microwave

Replace plastic with glass, metal, iron, bamboo, and wood.

estrogen-free.com

LEVEL 2

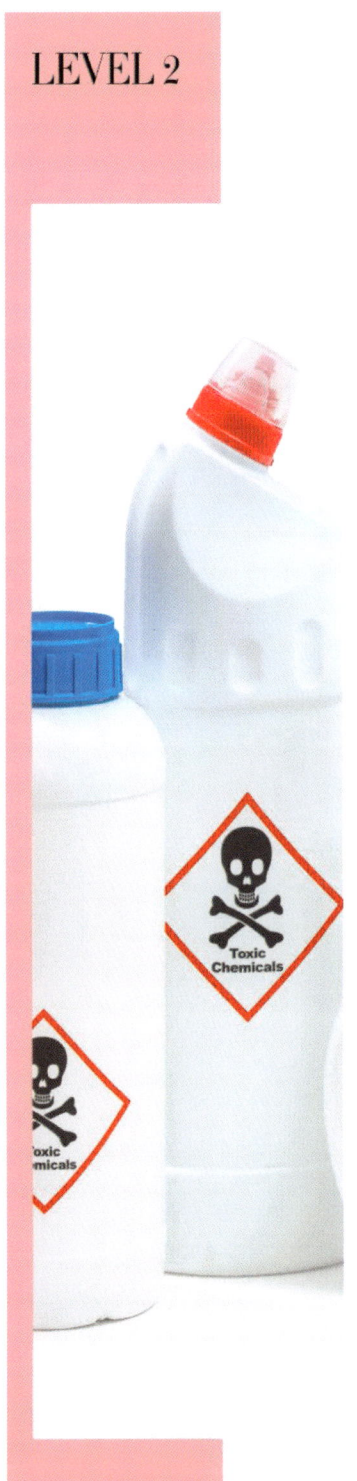

Avoid synthetic estrogens or xenoestrogens and chemicals in skincare and household items:

- All antibacterial products
- Chemical skincare products (e.g., Neutrogena moisturizer, cleanser, serums, sunscreens)
- Chemical bath and body products (e.g., Dial soap, bath wash, lotion, deodorant)
- Chemical laundry detergent, fabric softener, and dryer sheets (e.g., Tide)
- Chemical hair care products (e.g., Head and Shoulders shampoo, conditioner, hairspray, gels)
- Hand sanitizer and wipes containing Triclosan
- Perfume
- Scented products, candles (except beeswax), and air fresheners
- Toothpaste with fluoride and detergents
- 4-MBC (4-Methylbenzylidene camphor) in sunscreen lotions
- Alkylphenols (intermediate chemicals used in manufacturing)
- BPA and BPA-free hazardous alternatives BPS, BPAF, and TMBPF
- BHA (butylated hydroxyanisole) as a food preservative
- Insecticides (e.g., DDT, dieldrin, endosulfan)
- Parabens in lotions
- PCBs (polychlorinated biphenyls) formerly used in electrical oils, lubricants, adhesives, paints
- Pentachlorophenol (restricted general biocide and wood preservative)
- Phthalates and DEHP (plasticizers)
- Propyl gallate (used to protect oils and fats in products from oxidation)
- Nonylphenol and derivatives (industrial surfactants, emulsifiers)
- Metalloestrogens (a class of inorganic xenoestrogens)

estrogen-free.com

LEVEL 2

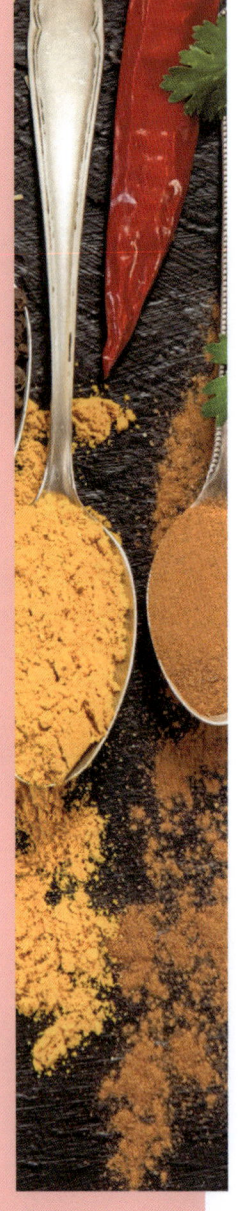

Avoid supplements containing these herbs:

- Aloe (A. barbadensis Mill., Aloe indica Royle)
- Ashwagandha/Indian ginseng (Withania somnifera)
- Asian ginseng (Panax ginseng, Ren shen)
- Astragalus/Huang qi (Astragalus membranaceus)
- Bitter Melon seeds (Momordica charantia)
- Black cohosh (Cimicifuga racemosa, Sheng ma)
- Black seed (Nigella sativa)
- Burdock root (Arctium lappa)
- Chasteberry (Vitex agnuscastus)
- Chinese moss (Huperzia serrata)
- Dandelion/Pu Gong Ying (Taraxacum Mongolicum)
- Dong Gui/Dong Quai (Angelica sinensis)
- Fennel seeds (Foeniculum vulgare)
- Fenugreek (Trigonella foenum-graecum)
- Fo-Ti/Ye Jiao Teng (Polygonum multiflorum)
- Fructus cnidii monnieri (She chuang zi)
- Heartwood (PterocarpusSoyauxii)
- Hemp/CBD (Cannabis)
- Golden root/goldenseal or Siberian rhodiola (Rhodiola rosea)
- Hops (Humulus lupulus)
- Kudzu root (Pueraria montana)
- Lavender (Lavandula angustifolia, L. officinalis)
- Licorice (Glycyrrhiza glabra, Gan cao)
- Neem oil (Azadirachta indica)
- North American ginseng (Panax quinquefolius, Xi Yang Shen)
- Milk thistle (Silybum marianum)
- Mistletoe (Viscum album)
- Moringa seeds (Moringa oleifera)
- Mucuna (Astraptes fulgerator)
- Prickly pear/Nopal cactus (Opuntia)
- Resveratrol
- Red clover (Trifolium pratense)
- Red pine needle (Pinus resinosa)
- Rhubarb (Rheum rhabarbarum)
- Saw palmetto (Sabal fructus)
- Siberian Rhodiola (Rhodiola rosea)
- Stinging nettle (Urtica dioica)
- Tu Fu ling (Cornus officinalis)
- Turmeric (Curcuma longa)
- White Kwao Krua (Pueraria Candollei var. Mirifica)
- Xiang fu (Rhizoma cyperi rotundi)

Supplements should be used short-term as needed. Do not use long-term unless under the care of a trained herbalist, Ayurvedic, or Chinese medical physician.

LEVEL 3: LIMIT WEAKER PHYTOESTROGENS

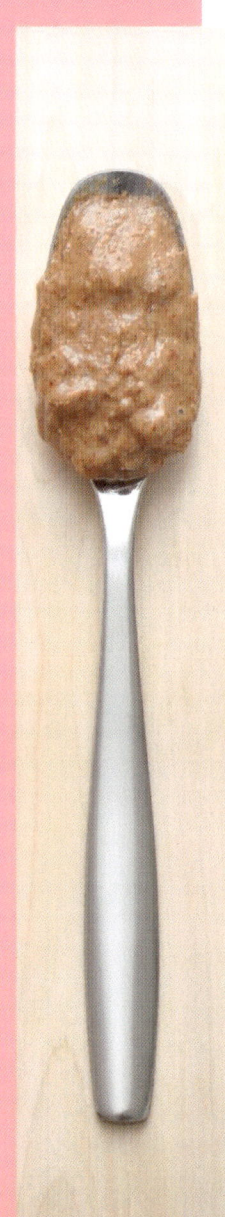

Limit these weaker phytoestrogens by consuming them in moderation. They are acceptable as long as they are not a staple in your diet. For example, drinking almond milk, eating almond butter, and using almond flour several times a week is excessive. Instead, incorporate them into a balanced diet by eating a handful of raw almonds a couple of times a week. ER+ breast cancer patients can eat, but in moderation.

Weaker Phytoestrogens:
- Sweet potatoes
- Oats, oatmeal, oat milk, oat flour
- Almond milk, almond butter, almond flour
- Chestnut flour, chestnut butter
- Grains
- Muesli
- Dried apricots
- Alfalfa sprouts
- Mung bean and sprouts
- Dried dates
- Dried prunes
- Figs
- Rye bread
- Winter squash
- Collard greens
- White beans
- Black bean sauce

Consume seeds in moderation and avoid concentrated supplements or seed cycling as large amounts can increase estrogen levels.

Limit Seeds:
- Hemp seeds
- Pumpkin seeds
- Sunflower seeds
- Walnuts
- Almonds
- Cashews
- Peanut butter
- Hazelnuts

estrogen-free.com

LEVEL 4: HOUSEHOLD ITEMS

Consider starting your journey to reduce toxicity and harmful xenoestrogens by gradually swapping out everyday household items. Small, consistent changes—like choosing natural bedding and non-toxic air fryers—can have a big impact on your health and well-being.

Everything we come into contact with daily in our homes contains chemicals: furniture, mattresses, bedding, pillows, rugs, flooring, toothbrushes, waterpiks, floss, washcloths, towels, toilet seats, bathtubs, showers, dinnerware, cups, utensils, ice trays, storage containers, air fryers, coffee makers, blenders, pots, pans, skillets, grills, and more. Even when we buy grass-fed organic products, they're often wrapped in plastic. We live in a chemical-driven society.

Avoid:
- Non-organic clothing, especially underwear
- Outgas non-organic clothing or buy used clothes
- Non-organic sheets, bedding, mattresses, towels, wash cloths, toothbrushes, hair brushes, and combs
- Vinyl flooring, carpet, rugs, furniture
- Outgas paint, carpet, furniture, mattresses, and fiberboard
- Plastic children's toys, bottles, diapers, pacifiers, and teething rings
- Pesticides - gardens, lawns, produce and home

Transform your home into a sanctuary for true wellness!

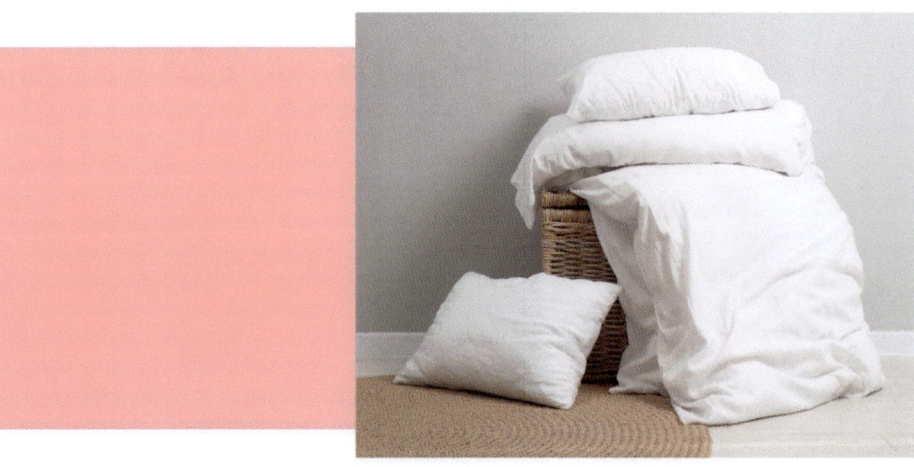

estrogen-free.com

LEVEL 5: DIY & GROW YOUR OWN

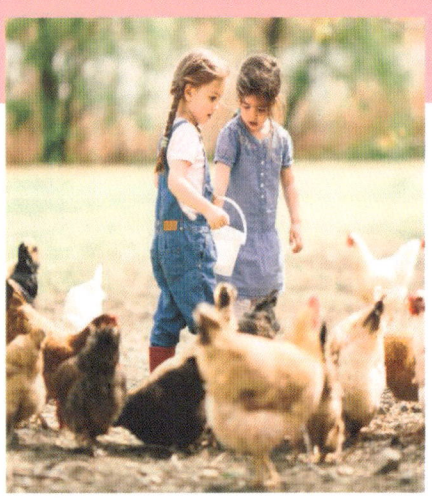

By following these guidelines and gradually replacing items as needed, you can create a healthier, estrogen-free environment that supports overall well-being and healthy hormones.

- Make most of your skincare and household items yourself
- Start growing some of your own food.

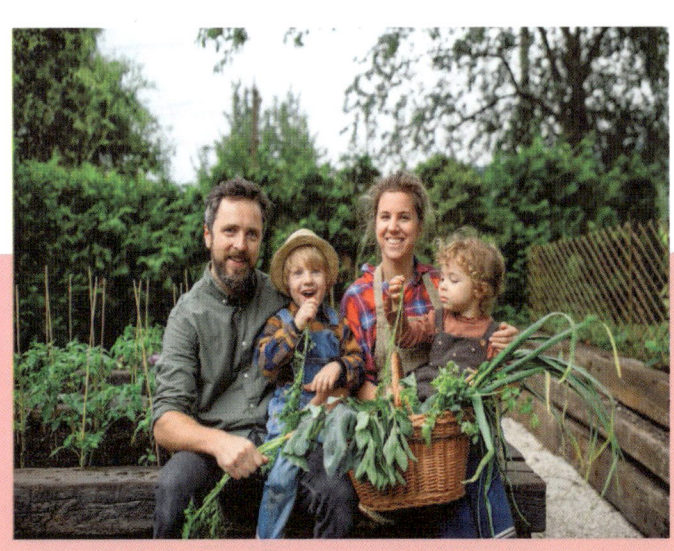

estrogen-free.com

UNLOCK THE SECRET TO PERMANENT HORMONE BALANCE

The ultimate key to hormone balance: treat the root cause by removing estrogen.

Hormone imbalances are not something you have to live with. The truth? The root cause of most hormonal issues is excess estrogen. It's time to address it head-on.

Just like with the Birth Control Pill, it takes about a year for your body to naturally metabolize excess estrogen. Yes, a year—but this process is worth it! Be patient, because this is how you create a strong foundation for lifelong hormone balance.

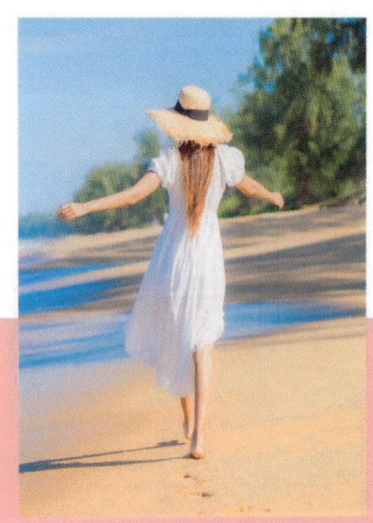

Here's what you need to know:
- Once your body has metabolized the excess estrogen, the key to staying balanced is simple: don't reintroduce it. That means being mindful of what you eat, drink, and use in your daily life.
- There is no supplement that can reduce estrogen. In fact, most supplements claiming to eliminate estrogen are actually phytoestrogens.
- The best part? Your body is not designed to produce excess estrogen on its own, so you don't need to worry about your body overproducing it. The real challenge is steering clear of external estrogen contaminants.

You have the power to take control of your hormone health. For answers to every question or myth you've heard about estrogen, check out the links on the next page.

Step into your power—arm yourself with knowledge and turn your hormone health goals into reality.

estrogen-free.com

BEING ESTROGEN FREE® IS THE NEW HEALTHY ALTERNATIVE

This is just a short guide to get you started. There's plenty more information available in other books, websites, blogs, and videos. For daily tips and reminders, follow on Instagram. For in-depth, uncensored research, information, and answers to all your questions, subscribe to The Boob Tube: Breast Thermography Research, Breast Cancer prevention and Your Guide to Becoming Your Own Hormone Specialist.

Quick Review:
• Avoid hormone specialists and doctors
• Avoid hormone protocols, treatments, and fads
• Avoid "women's" or "breast" treatments, supplements, herbs, and essential oils
• Avoid boobie butters or treatments for breast congestion
• Avoid supplements and herbal formulas unless prescribed for your specific health issue

Become a Boobie Activist—you can change the world, one breast at a time. Share the Estrogen Free® Lifestyle with your bestie, mother, sister, kids, and husband or partner.

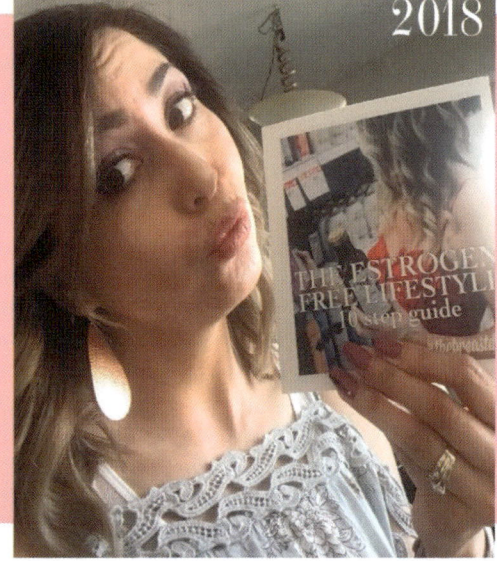

estrogen-free.com

Researched & written by Dr. Wendy

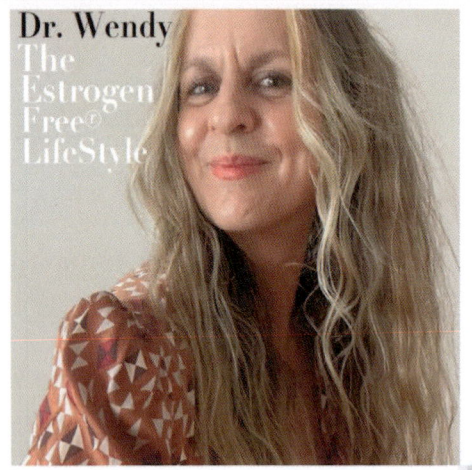

Dr. Wendy

THE ESTROGEN FREE® LIFESTYLE

ABOUT DR. WENDY

Wendy Sellens is a Chinese medical doctor, and a leading researcher in breast thermography and bio-identical hormones. She is president of the consumer advocacy group the Women's Academy of Breast Thermography, president of The Pink Bow Breast Thermography Research and Education non-profit, author of eight books including "Breast Thermography Revolution" and creator of the Estrogen Free® lifestyle to reduce risk of hormonal disorders in the entire family.

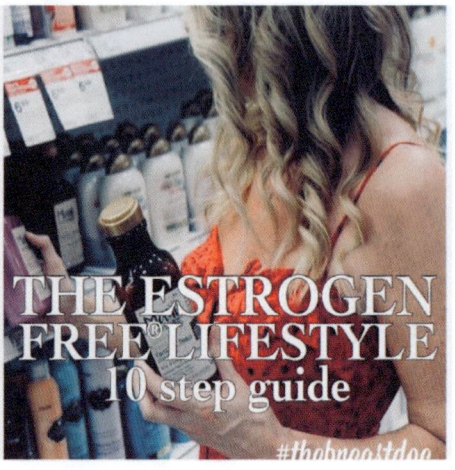

ELSEWHERE

www.estrogen-free.com
www.abreastboutique.com
www.estrogenfreecourses.com
www.mypinkimage.com
support@estrogen-free.com

Instagram: @estrogenfree
Twitter: @thebreastdoc
Facebook: womensacademybreastthermography

PRESS & PUBLICATIONS

8 Books
Courses & Certifications
Fox News
Local News, Newspapers & Magazines
"Cancer Free-Are You Sure?" Jenny Hrbacek RN
Radios Shows & Podcasts
Conferences
Merocla
Weston A. Price Journal

Printed in Dunstable, United Kingdom